YOU ARE WHAT YOU EAT

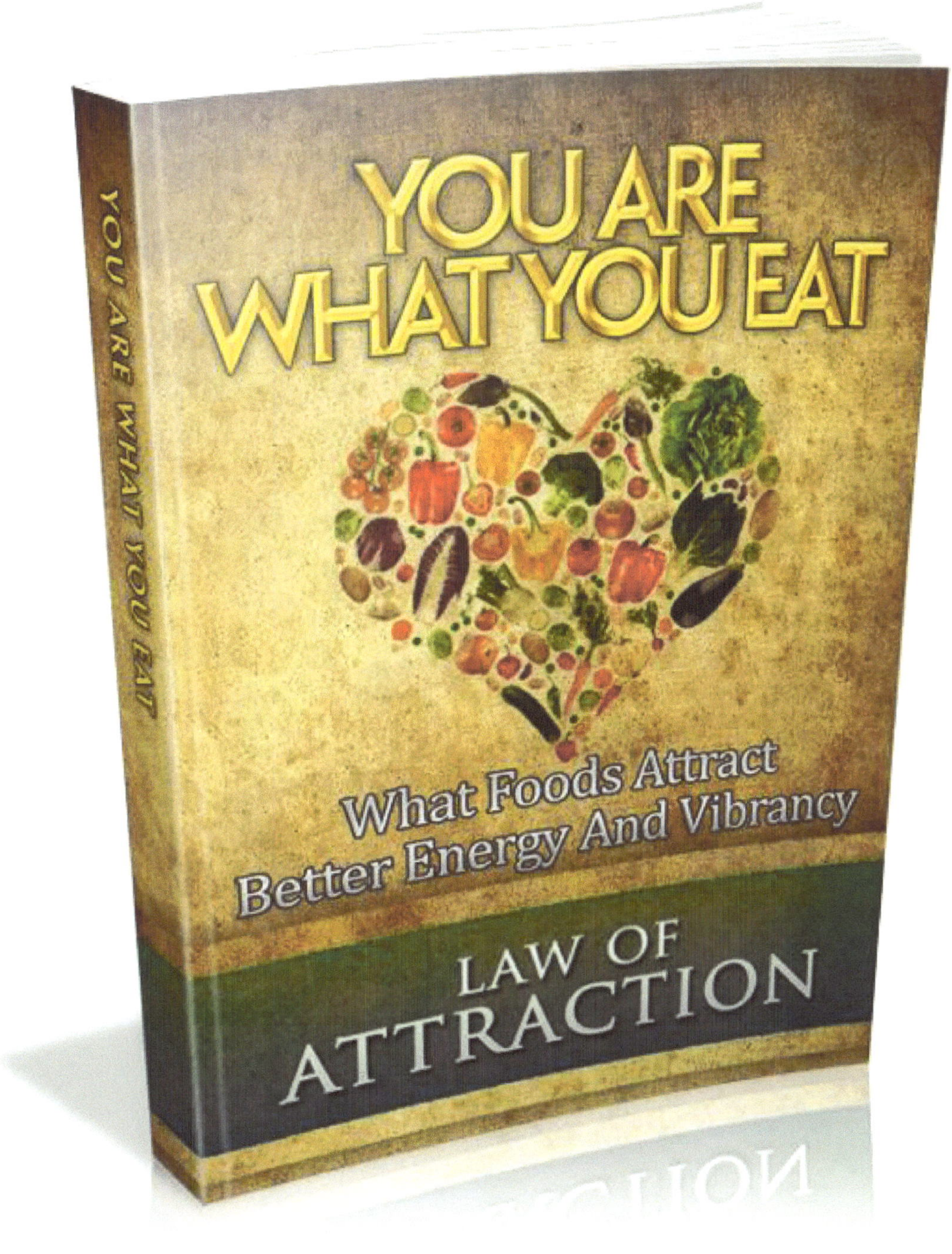

What Foods Attract Better Energy And Vibrancy

LAW OF ATTRACTION

Published ~ ©2012

Terms and Conditions

LEGAL NOTICE

The Publisher has strived to be as accurate and complete as possible in the creation of this report, notwithstanding the fact that he does not warrant or represent at any time that the contents within are accurate due to the rapidly changing nature of the Internet.

While all attempts have been made to verify information provided in this publication, the Publisher assumes no responsibility for errors, omissions, or contrary interpretation of the subject matter herein. Any perceived slights of specific persons, peoples, or organizations are unintentional.

In practical advice books, like anything else in life, there are no guarantees of income made. Readers are cautioned to reply on their own judgment about their individual circumstances to act accordingly.

This book is not intended for utilize as a source of legal, business, accounting or financial advice. All readers are advised to seek services of competent professionals in legal, business, accounting and finance fields.

You are encouraged to print this book for easy reading.

Table Of Contents

Foreword

Nutrition makes up a large portion of you health and appearance. Many professionals will testify that as much as 80% of your weight loss and fitness results are based on your diet.

This means that you could exercise all throughout the day, but if you're eating unhealthy food, your body will surely show it.

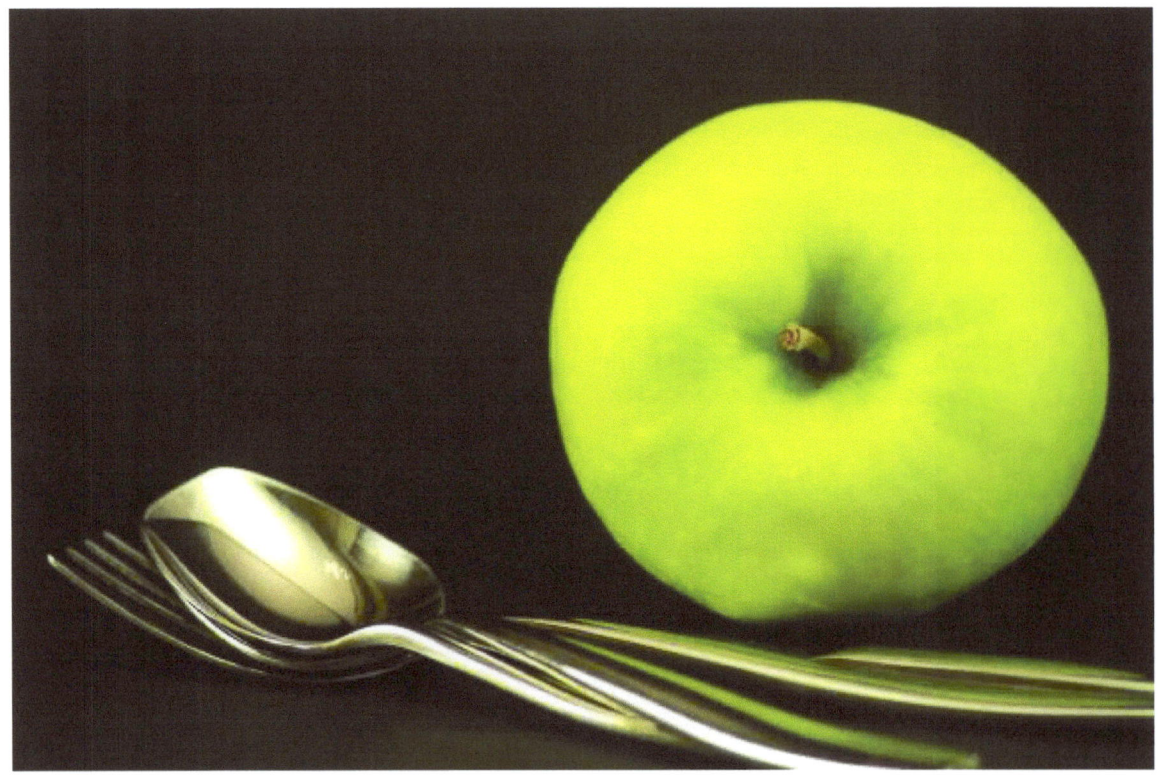

Law Of Attraction: You Are What You Eat

What Foods Attract Better Energy And Vibrancy.

Chapter 1:

About Nutrition

Synopsis

Nutrition is a matter that people spend their careers learning about and requires volumes of books to explain. My objective is to instruct you how to consume a healthy nutritional diet that aids your body in burning off fat instead of storing it. You do not require overwhelming science to "get" this.

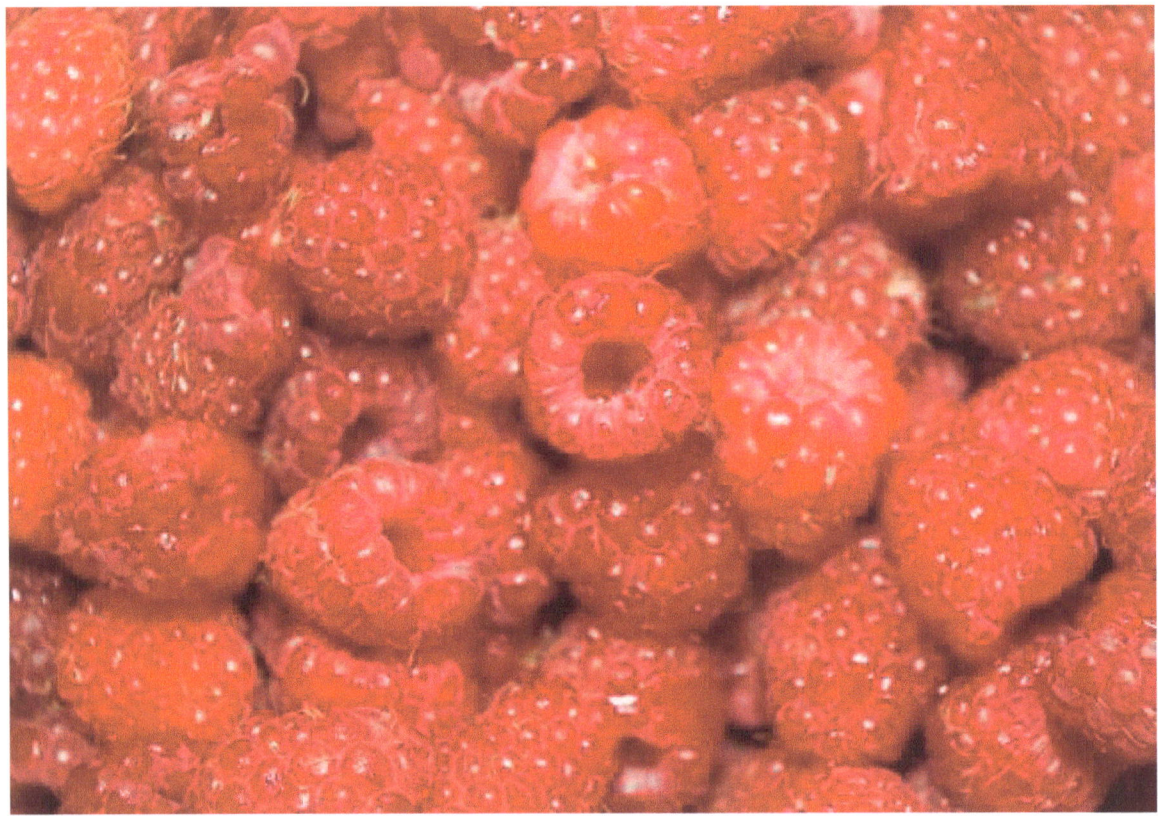

Published ~ ©2012

What It's About

A healthy nutritional diet requires being well rounded with the suitable amount of nutrients, vitamins as well as minerals. The RDA's recommendation for day-to-day consumption of such things is a good place to check your optimal intakes.

The first thing that you should know about nutrition is this information: Consuming little meals every few hours will boost your metabolism and reduce fat storage. This is a proven fact that muscle-builders, models, athletes and thin people generally follow - you should give it a try as well.

Consuming the proper foods once you wake up is critical when breaking the fast your body goes into nightly. Approximately 3-4 hours after you eat your body shuts down your metabolism and behaves as though it is required to store food. This is a great function to possess if a shortage erupts and you do not see food for a long period of time. After all, if there is a shortage you're going to need your body to work "efficiently" by stashing away fat, and burning it as little as possible.

Nevertheless, you don't desire your body to stock up on fat and burn it slowly now, correct? Because there's no food shortage or famine at the time being (and more than likely wont be one in the near future) then it's pretty irritating when your body begins loading up on the pounds. So, in order to communicate with your body that it's fit, well-nourished, and not in demand of additional fat storage you need to reprogram your metabolism.

Here's the way you do it. Begin your day off with a little meal and continue to eat small meals every few hours throughout the day.

What should you eat? Here I'm simply going to give you general guidelines - because we would have to sit down together to make a precise fat burning diet plan for your body. These suggestions are a basic guideline to healthy types of food that don't boost fat storage.

- ➢ Protein: 35%
- ➢ Fat: 25%
- ➢ Carbs: 40%
- ➢

All meals that you eat should contain calories coming from protein, carbs and fat. Your body is required to consume each of these in small portions throughout the day - as you take in a meal that's 90% carbohydrate 5% fat and 5% protein your body is going to digest it quicker (i.e. feel hungry again quicker) even if the calorie count is the same as a meal with above percentages, and you have more potential to stash away a percentage of the carbs as fat.

Hang on...

Do not go and get rid of the carbs out of your meals quite yet. Trimming down carbs could cause your body to once more enter fat storage mode. Trust me, you don't need that.

Chapter 2:

Why Eat Well

Synopsis

Eating healthy food is important at all ages, but it's particularly important as you get older. For numerous adults however, consuming healthy food day in and day out can be a bit rough. Why should I eat well? What is the link between consuming healthy food and maturing well? What may I do to eat healthier? How can I choose realistic goals that I am capable of meeting?

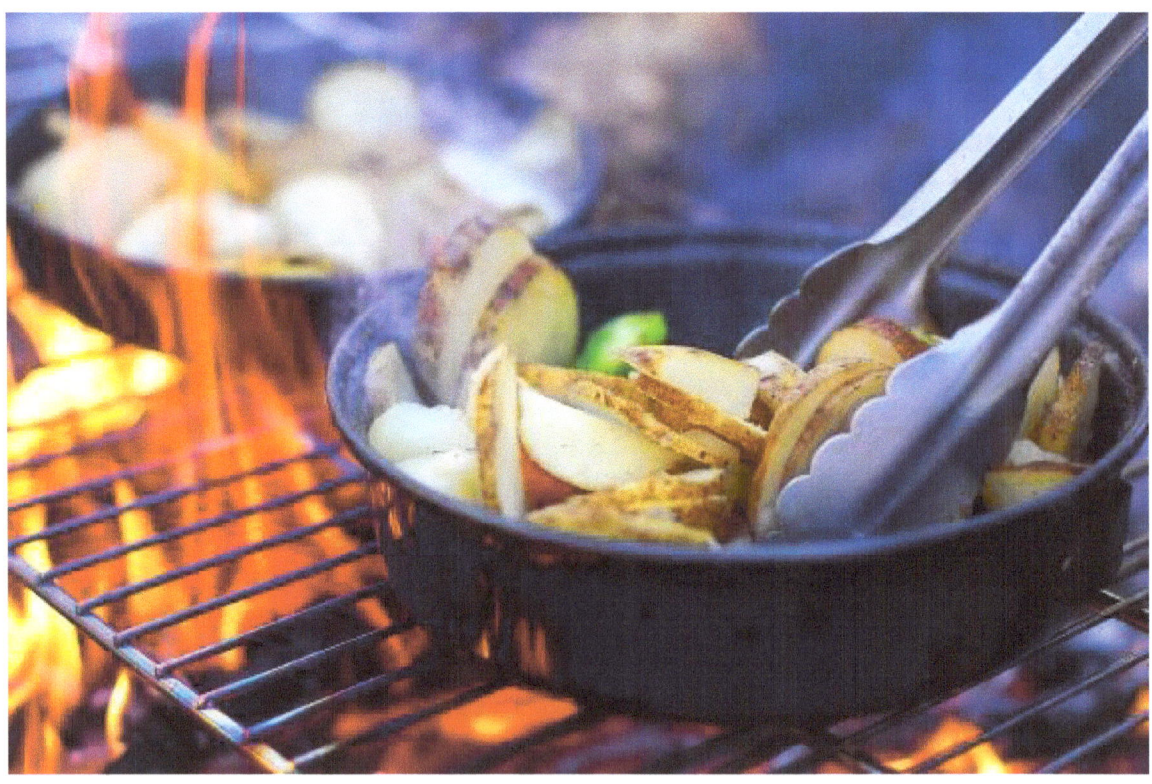

The Reasoning

Why do I need to eat healthy food?

Regardless of when you begin, eating a healthy diet can assist you in maintaining and even improving your health - even more so if you combine it with exercise as well.

Putting together, healthy eating habits and routine physical activity can be the difference between independence and a life of being able to do nothing on your own.

This can aid you in life by providing you with the energy you require to remain active and do the things you wish to do. As well, healthy eating can also stop or slow down the advancement of numerous chronic sicknesses, such as heart disease and diabetes, osteoporosis and a few types of cancer. Eating healthy can also help you deal better with both physical and mental strain, operations and even the common cold or influenza.

What is the link between consuming healthy food and maturing well?

Healthy living - which includes both consuming healthy food and maintaining a regular exercise routine - can assist you in conforming to the natural maturing process and keep your youthful vigor.

The fundamentals of healthy living:

Consume an assortment of foods. Eat in moderation. Size matters, so limit your portions!

Consume a lot of:

> Veggies and fruit
> Whole grains (for example, breads, pasta, oatmeal and brown rice)
> Legumes (such as dried beans, peas, lentils)
> Sea Food
> Unsaturated fats (from vegetable oils, nuts, and seeds)
> Lean meat (for example chicken and turkey)

Consume Less:

> Saturated fats (found in butter, lard, deli meats, bacon and
> sausages)
> Trans fats (found in processed foods, cookies, cakes and deep-fried foods)
> Refined or enriched grains
> Salt and sugar (including sugary drinks as well as jams, candies
> and baked goods)

> Consume a lot of water.
> Participate in something active daily.

What am I able to do to consume better food?

The difficult part is to eat in a fashion that aids you in maintaining a healthy weight, while also providing you with the nutrients you require for good health.

> Veggies and fruit

 Published ~ ©2012

- ➢ Grain products, including bread rice, pasta and cereals
- ➢ Milk and alternatives like low fat cheese and yogurt
- ➢ Meat - fish, shellfish, poultry, lean meat - and alternatives, like eggs, beans, lentil, chickpeas, tofu and nuts.

How am I able to determine goals that I can in reality accomplish?

The simplest method to move towards consuming healthy food daily is to set goals that you truly can meet. For instance, say to yourself:

- ➢ I'll eat one more fruit and one more veggie today.
- ➢ I'll try a fruit or vegetable this week that I have never tried before.
- ➢ I'll eat fish once this week.
- ➢ I'll choose whole grain bread for my sandwich.
- ➢ I'll drink one more glass of water each day.
- ➢ I'll be more active today.
- ➢ I'll throw out my deep fryer.
- ➢ I'll do most of my shopping around the outer edges of the grocery store, because that's where the fresh foods are.

A couple of small changes can rise up to a very big difference to your health - before you even know its happening!

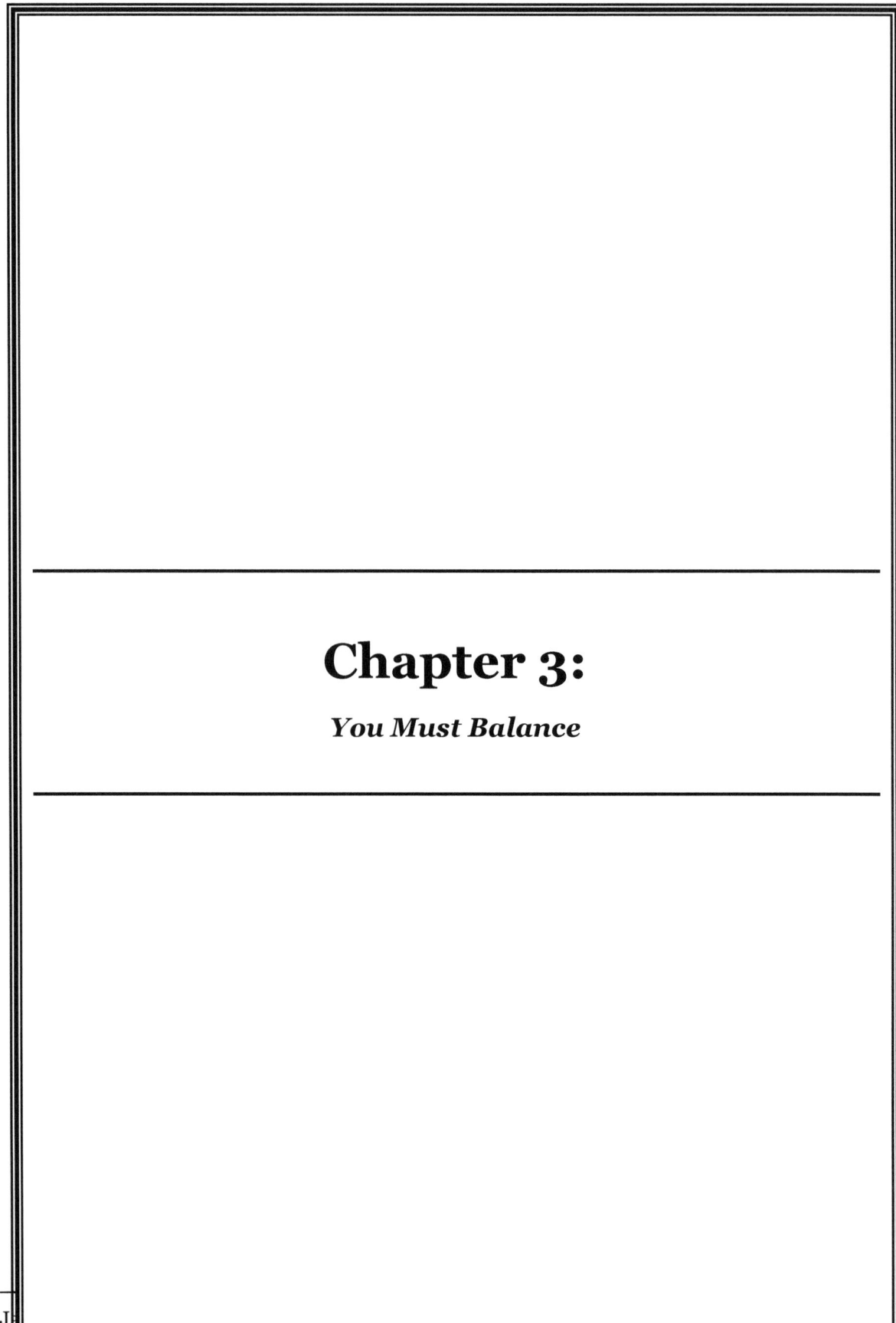

Chapter 3:

You Must Balance

Synopsis

Balance is everything? What is healthy food? It looks so perplexing. Is there a simple method to make certain I acquire all the nutrients I need? Alright, I understand the four food groups. However what's a proper portion? How come veggies and fruits are so crucial? What about coffee, tea and alcoholic beverages? What about salt? Are organic foods healthier for me? Where does exercising fit in?

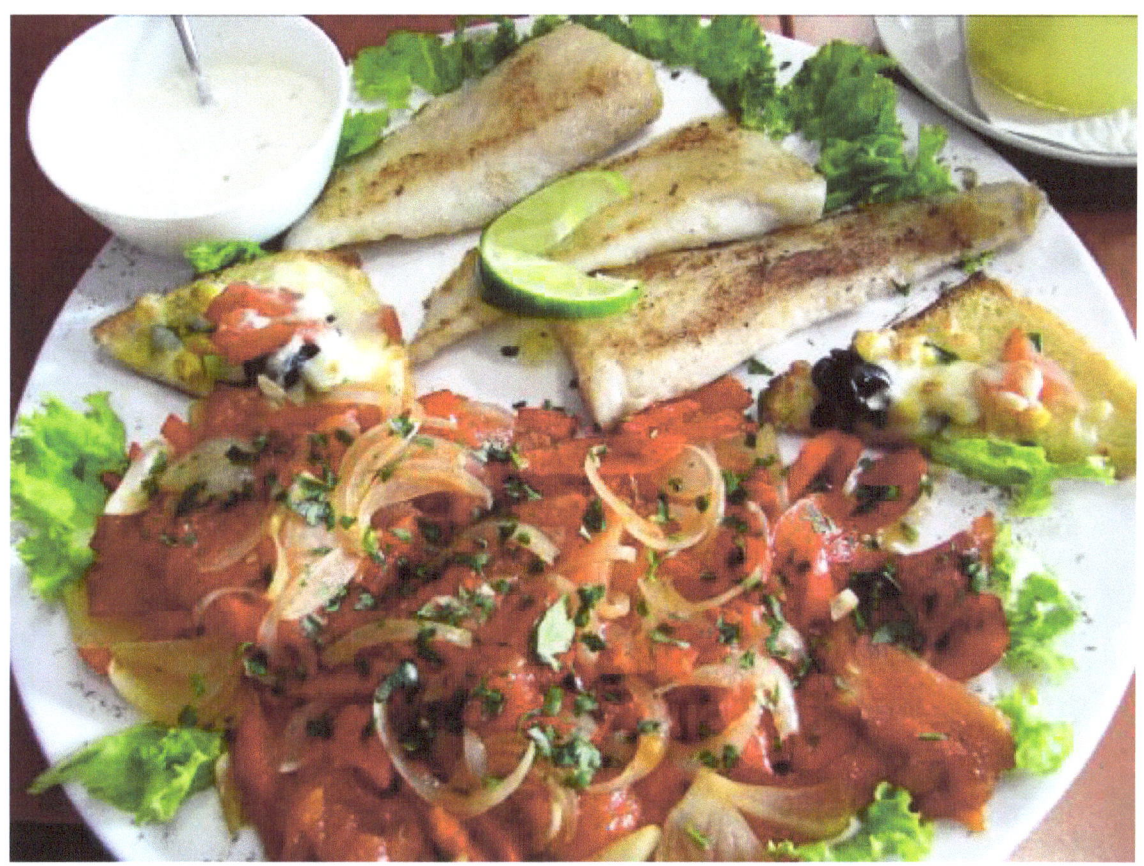

     Published ~ ©2012

Adjusting

A nutrient is a substance that supplies nourishment necessary for life and growth. Eating healthy food is a significant method to make certain you acquire all the nutrients you need, with no additional calories or additional weight gain. If what you're eating doesn't provide you with adequate nutrition, you are able to take a multivitamin/mineral and/or other supplements to assist

What is healthy eating?
Healthy eating is balanced eating, where you eat an assortment of foods. It includes protein, carbs (especially fiber), fats and fluids.

Protein
Protein helps restore your muscular tissue, skin and nails. It can assist you in healing yourself if you have been sick or have had an operation. The greatest sources of protein include meat, fish, poultry, milk, eggs, cheese, yogurt, legumes (dried peas, beans and lentils for instance), nuts, seeds and soy products (tofu or soy beverages for instance).Whole grains, veggies and fruit can also supply little amounts of protein.

Here's how you are able to simply acquire the protein your body requires daily along with a lot of other good nutrients, like iron, calcium and vitamin B12:

> In the morning, consume a few egg whites as well as a piece of whole wheat toast and a banana. You can also try some oatmeal made with a few egg whites and milk or unsweetened, fortified soy beverage, or dry cereal make with low-fat buttermilk.

- ➢ In the afternoon, eat a piece of low fat cheese and some lentil soup. You might also want to try steamed brown rice with cut-up chicken chunks and veggies like green beans or bok choy.

- ➢ When snack time comes around, consume a handful of nuts with three-quarters of a cup of low-fat yogurt, or a little cup of milk or unsweetened, fortified soy beverage.

- ➢ At supper time, eat sea food (or tofu) with half a cup of brown or basmati rice, and half a cup of broccoli or other veggies and one cup of assorted salad.

Attempt to have a good source of protein at every meal. Try:
- ➢ Adding a piece of low fat cheese to your preferred sandwich
- ➢ Chopping up a hard-boiled egg and putting it into your salad
- ➢ Consuming a handful of unsalted soy nuts
- ➢ Scattering nuts and seeds on your cereal, salad or stir fry
- ➢ Scattering natural almond butter on a piece of whole wheat toast or a whole wheat tortilla
- ➢ Placing chickpeas or beans into a stir fry or pasta sauce.
- ➢ If you're still having difficulty acquiring sufficient protein through your eating habits, take a protein shake daily.

Carbs

Healthy carbs - like veggies, fruit, whole grains and low-fat dairy products - supply your body with the fuel your heart, lungs and additional organs need to operate properly. They have essential vitamins and minerals and assist you by giving you the energy you require to run another lap, swim a bit longer or to do an additional set of weight-lifts. Several are also crucial sources of fiber. A couple of carbs, nevertheless, are unhealthy- especially the ones that are easy to digest and that rapidly raise your blood sugar. These include white bread, white rice, cookies and cakes.

A few weight loss plans tell you to cut back on or get rid of all carbs since they make you put on more weight. Only that seriously restricts what you are able to consume and you lose out on numerous crucial nutrients.

Fiber

The majority of adults get only about 50% of the fiber they should be consuming every day. Fiber is a nutrient obtained from plants. In order to keep your bowels regular and healthy you are required to consume fiber. Consuming several high-fiber foods can also assist you to lower your blood cholesterol levels, maintain blood sugar levels and aid in preventing high blood pressure. Since fiber curves your appetite for longer periods of time, it can aid with weight control as well.

Grains and grain products are especially high in fiber levels. In reality, a high-fiber cereal for breakfast (one with four grams or more of fiber) will assist you in keeping your hunger in check for the entire day. Follow up throughout the day with additional high-fiber foods, like whole wheat toast or pasta with vegetable sauce, a hot bowl of chili, or low-fat yogurt with fruit and bran sprinkled on top. Fruits and veggies, beans, lentils and chickpeas are also excellent sources or fiber.

Fats

Studies now show that it's not fat that's unhealthy for you, but rather the kind of fat you consume that matters most. Everybody requires some fat to remain healthy. Fat supplies your body with vitality and aids in constructing a protective coat around your cells -but it must be healthy fat and in the correct portions.

Fats to avoid are saturated and trans fats. Saturated fats are generally discovered in food that came from animals. Trans fats come generally from vegetable oils that have been made solid by a method named hydrogenation.

Unhealthy fats are found in:
- ➢ Whole or full - fat milk
- ➢ Cream, sour cream as well as ice cream
- ➢ Butter as well as clarified butter
- ➢ Cheese
- ➢ Fatty red meat (sausage, pork bacon, Chinese preserved meats)
- ➢ Chicken, duck as well as turkey skin of fat
- ➢ Hard margarines as well as vegetable shortening
- ➢ Partially hydrogenated vegetable oil
- ➢ Deep-fried foods
- ➢ Baked items (including cookies, cakes, pies and pastries)

Healthy fat are found in:
- ➢ Oily or fatty fish, such as salmon, anchovies, rainbow trout, sardines, mackerel, char and herring
- ➢ Nuts and seeds, such as cashews, almonds, walnuts, peanuts, and ground flaxseeds
- ➢ Vegetable oils, including olive, peanut, canola, soybean, and sesame oil
- ➢ Flaxseed as well as walnut oils (do not heat these oils; utilize them cold)
- ➢ Wheat germ
- ➢ Avocadoes

Foods strengthened with omega 3, including eggs, yogurt as well as soy beverage.

To make certain you're consuming the correct portion of fat, begin by picking foods that are naturally low in fat, and then add no more than two to three tablespoons (30 to 45 grams) of healthy, unsaturated fats to what you eat daily. This includes oil utilized for making food, salad dressings, margarine and mayonnaise.

As well, try to replace healthy fat for unhealthy fat wherever you are able to, and remember to study food labels cautiously. Low fat means that the food has less than three grams of fat per serving. Fat free means that the food has less than 0.5 grams of fat per serving.

Additionally:
> Choose lean meats, and then trim off all fat you are able to see.
> Take off the skin from chicken as well as turkey.
> Grill, broil or roast your meat, chicken or turkey to allow the fat to drain off.
> Eat fish two or more times a week.
> Choose legumes instead of meat at least once a week. Cook a dish that utilizes baked beans, lentils or chickpeas, or prepare a batch of chili.
> Cook with low-fat dairy products made with skim or 1% milk of yogurt.
> Utilize low-fat milk in your coffee and tea.
> Utilize some mustard, ketchup, relish, cranberry sauce, or natural almond butter instead of butter or margarine.
> Choose a healthy, low-fat salad dressing or create your own.

Chapter 4:

Salt and Veggies

Published ~ ©2012

Synopsis

How come veggies and fruits so crucial? Researchers have recognized for a while that veggies and fruits are full of matters that are critical to health, such as fiber, vitamin C and E and other antioxidants. Nowadays, new research is discovering that there are even more beneficial things hidden inside apples and green beans.

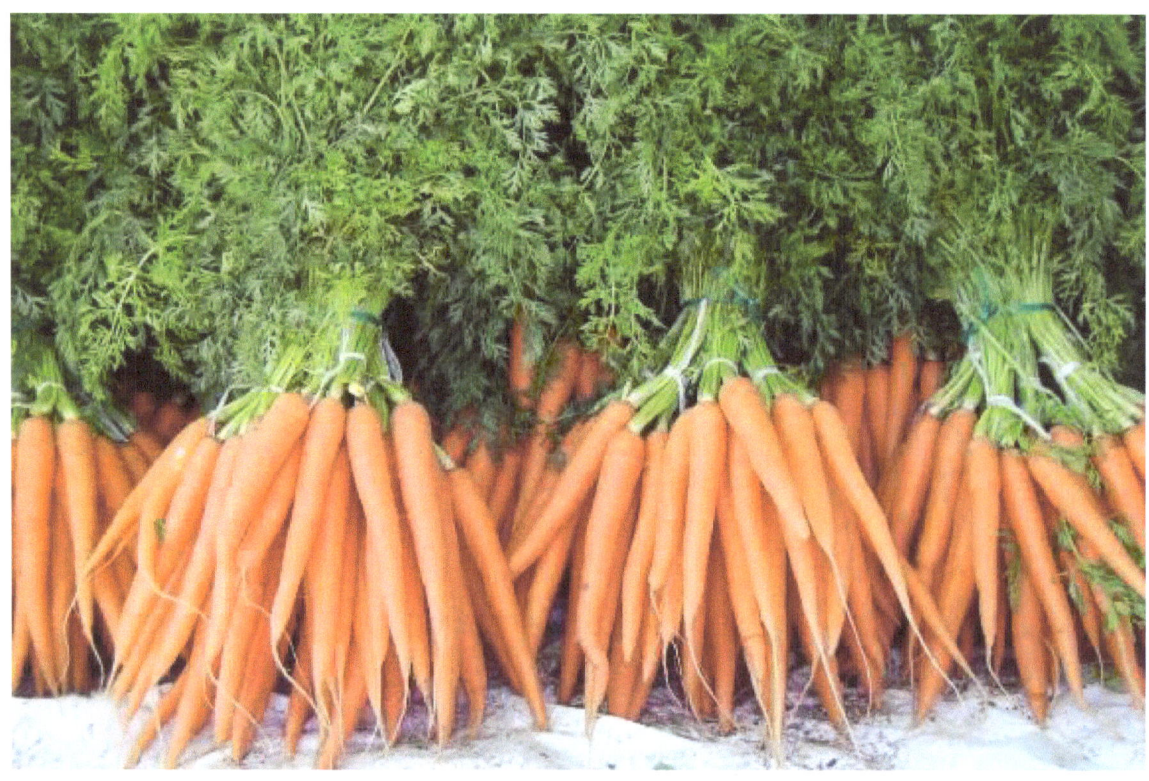

Important Info

Phytochemicals are chemicals brought forth by plants. These chemicals carry compounds that might protect against disease, particularly cancer, and perhaps osteoporosis and eye disease.

The brightest and most colorful vegetables and fruits - the dark green, orange, yellow and red ones - are jammed with both necessary vitamins and minerals and disease-fighting phytochemicals. Soy products, beans and lentils, as well, are full of phytochemicals - so remember to include them. And do not be concerned about seasoning your foods with herbs, spices and citrus peels to get additional nutrients.

What about salt?
You more than likely know that consuming an excessive amount of sodium (salt) may increase blood pressure, which may lead to heart disease. Only recent research exposes that the effects of high blood pressure are even more varied.

Investigators now recognize that high blood pressure may also accelerate the body's loss of calcium, which could lead to osteoporosis (thinning of the bones that cause them to break easily).High blood pressure is also believed to be a "risk factor" for diabetes and kidney disease, which implies you're more probable to acquire these diseases.

You should restrict your consumption of sodium to fewer than 2300 mgs per day (that is about one teaspoon of salt) from all your foods.

 Published ~ ©2012

You should eat even less sodium if you've got high blood pressure, osteoporosis, kidney disease or diabetes.

The most effective method to control your sodium consumption is to consume fresh vegetables and fruits more frequently and prepare your own food. Try not to rely on frozen dinners or canned soup, meat or vegetables, as most bear a great deal of excess salt. If you do however purchase these foods, search for labels that read "no salt added" or "low sodium." Just look out for labels that read "reduced sodium" or "less salt," since the food might still have a high amount of salt.

Low salt tips:
  ➤ Don't add salt while cooking
  ➤ While you're dining out, ask the cook to hold the salt.
  ➤ Remove the saltshaker off the dining table.
  ➤ Replace other seasonings for salt, like herbs, dry mustard, spices, lemon juice, ginger or garlic.
  ➤ Pick out fresh food as frequently as possible
  ➤ Avoid frozen dinners.
  ➤ Rinse off canned foods, like salmon, tuna fish and beans, under water to get rid of the salt.
  ➤ Avoid "instant" foods, including instant soups, oatmeal, pancakes and waffles.
  ➤ Avoid processed cheese.
  ➤ Avoid meats that have been processed, cured, or smoked.
  ➤ These include sausages, hot dogs, ham, bacon, pepperoni or smoked fish.
  ➤ Restrict snack foods, like salted crackers, chips, popcorn and salty nuts.

Chapter 5:

Slimming Down

Synopsis

What should I consume if I'm overweight?

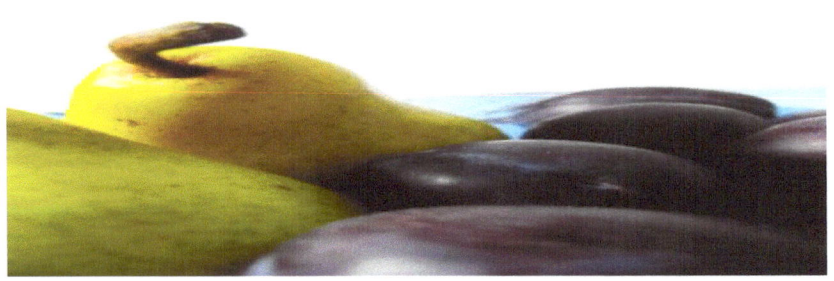

Lose It

A fit weight is the key to a healthy maturing.

You may put on weight because:

> ➤ You eat too many calories. Perhaps you're dining out several times a week, consuming portions that are too big, snacking too frequently on high-fat foods or consuming drinks that hold a lot of sugar.

> ➤ You're not active enough and inactive people are more plausible to carry extra amounts body fat.

> ➤ You're losing muscle and acquiring fat as your metabolism decelerates.

Since muscle assists in burning calories, you'll discover that it is more difficult to burn off what you consume. At the same time, your body requires fewer calories the more you age, even if you're active.

Variety is the key

Whenever you consume an assortment of different foods, you will not feel bored or deprived and you're more plausible to acquire all the nutrients you require.

Eat breakfast

Consuming breakfast is among the most crucial things you are able to do to lose weight.

During the nighttime, your metabolism decelerates. Consuming a balanced breakfast - like high-fiber cereal, fruit and milk - assists you to jump-start your body in the morning and it will burn fuel a lot more effectively throughout the day.

Plan our meals around high-fiber foods

You'll find you are less hungry if you consume additional vegetables, fruit, legumes (like beans, lentils and chickpeas), as well as whole grains. Always consume three meals and two to three snacks daily. Once you have skipped a meal or snack, you will often consume more at the next one too frequently.

Watch your fats

Since you require some fat to remain healthy, make certain you select healthy fats rather than unhealthy fats. Unhealthy fats are saturated and trans fats. Healthy fats include monounsaturated and polyunsaturated fats. They could really cut down your cholesterol levels and your chance for heart disease and stroke.

Healthy fats are found in vegetable oils, fish, nuts and seeds; even so, since nuts and seeds are as well high in calories, consume them in low amounts.

Only a couple of calories less a day...

To sustain your weight, you want to burn off the same amount of calories you consume. Merely a couple of additional calories daily can tip the balance. For instance, an additional one hundred calories daily sums up to ten pounds of additional weight by the end of a year. That is a piece of bread and margarine, one scoop of ice cream or one can of soda per day.

But if you are able to scratch out those additional calories, or do more to burn them up, there is no reason you can not keep up your weight or even drop off a couple of pounds. Clean out your cupboards and make the healthy selection the simple selection.

Control your portions

Just about all people underrate the amount of food they consume daily by as much as one-third. For instance, a portion of fresh veggies amounts to a half a cup of broccoli, one portion of grains amounts to a half a cup of brown rice or pasta, one portion of meat is two-and-a-half ounces of lean beef and so forth.

Select your fluids wisely

What you drink may be just as significant as what you consume. Only one soft drink daily can accumulate to ten pounds yearly.

Regular soft drinks, fruit juice and alcohol are all high in calories (soft drinks, particularly, can also add to tooth disintegration).

Even coffee and tea may be packed with calories if you add sugar, cream or whole milk. As well, fancy coffees, liked flavored lattes and cappuccinos, can be as calorie-rich as a piece of cake.

Wrapping Up

By taking the time to study this, you have stepped onto the route that leads to an in shape, healthy body. Take a minute to think over the famous quote ***"Success is a journey, not a destination".*** We may replace the word 'success' with the word 'fitness'.

Learning to make the correct decisions in your nutrition will convert to a lifestyle that is never ending.

As you relish a lowered body fat, high energy levels and your right body weight you will feel your self-confidence and health greatly gain. Begin to construct the habits that will step-up your enjoyment and quality of life today! I have every confidence that you will be able to bring in this a part of your life.

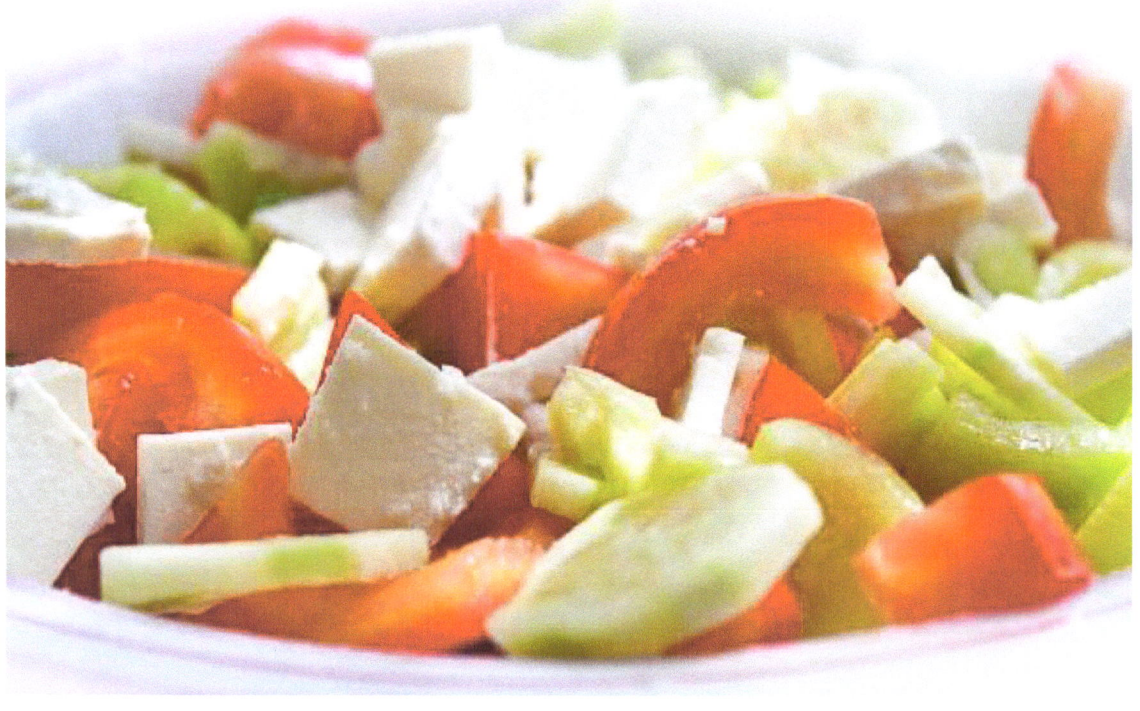